THIS COOKBOOK WILL SAVE YOUR LIFE

Amazing & Easy Flavorful Dash Recipes That Will Put Your Hearth in Great Shape

Fit Chef Dash

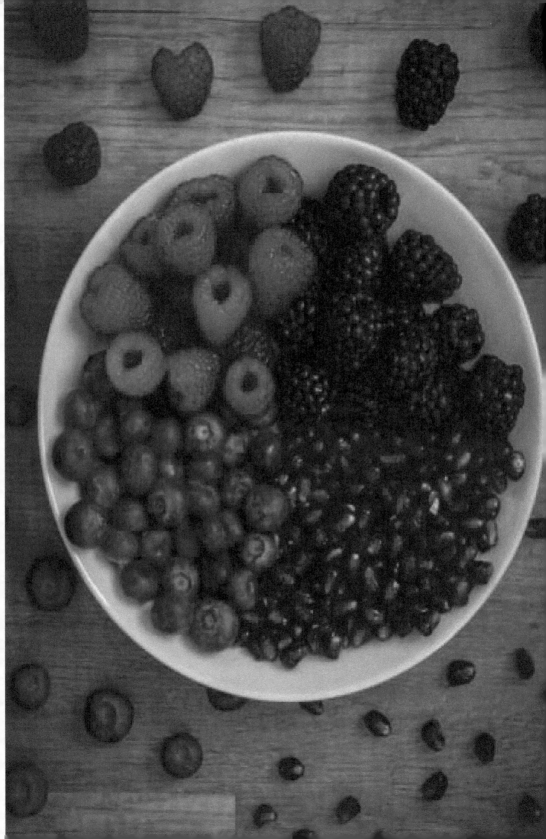

Table of Contents

INTRODUCTION

The Dash diet is a dietary approach to treat hypertension. It helps to maintain, improve, and support overall health as well as lowering blood pressure. The diet was created by the National Institute of Health as a way to treat hypertension without medication. The main idea of the Dash diet is to reduce the amount of sodium in food while eating nutrients that help to maintain normal blood pressure. These nutrients are calcium, potassium, and magnesium.

The Dash diet can give you awesome results in just two weeks. The nutrition plan is a scientifically proved system designed by physicians to reduce your blood pressure up to 15.

It also helps with weight loss and in preventing heart disease, cancer, osteoporosis, diabetes, and stroke. It is not a restrictive diet; it is a lifestyle that can be followed with very little adjustment. If your goal is weight loss, the Dash diet can be personalized by a nutritionist or doctor because its standard form wasn't designed for that purpose.

Dash Diet for Weight Loss and to Lower Blood Pressure

For the last few years, the Dash diet has been one of the highest-rated of the most popular diets. It has proven to be effective in fighting high blood pressure.

According to the National Institutes of Health, the success of the diet in weight loss is 3.3 points out of 5 and 4.8 points out of 5 in neutralizing and lowering blood pressure. The major cause of high blood pressure is dietary sodium. Excessive concentration of sodium leads to deposits in the blood vessel's walls. The chemical composition of sodium attracts water, which causes swelling and narrowing of the blood vessels. Therefore, the blood pressure rises and causes hypertension.

Studies suggested that, on average, during a 70-year lifespan, a person can eat approximately half a ton of salt. This is the only mineral that we eat in its pure form. It doesn't mean that salt is harmful to our bodies. Like every mineral, it has benefits and is imperative for regulating the water-salt balance in the body, the formation of gastric juice, and the transfer of oxygen in blood cells. However, when it is present in excessive amounts, it can be a disaster.

The Dash diet allows you to decrease the amount of sodium in your body. The recommended daily amount of sodium should not exceed 2300mg. Some studies show that reducing the amount of sodium to 1500mg can help to control high blood pressure.

The diet is balanced with nutrients that are very important for normal blood pressure, such as potassium, magnesium, calcium, protein, and plant fibers. The perfect combination of these nutrients will give remarkable results.

The Dash diet is the perfect combination of different food groups such as fruits, vegetables, grains, dairy products, meat, fish, poultry, eggs, nuts and seeds, legumes, and oils. In addition, you will consume less salt, sugar, and fatty foods, which are a cause of high blood cholesterol. If you follow the diet strictly and do physical activity every day, it is possible to lose 17-19 lbsin4 months.

The major advantage of dash eating is that it is based on the body's natural eating patterns. And the lost weight doesn't return if you adopt it as a lifestyle. The dash diet is considered one of the healthiest diets. Although it was created for hypertensive patients, it can improve the well-being and health of anyone.

What to Eat and Avoid on Dash Diet:

Grains

In this diet, you can have whole-grains, which are rich in fiber and nutrients. It is easy to find low-fat versions to substitute for the high-fat choices.

What to Eat	Eat Occasionally	What to avoid
Whole grain breakfast cereals	Whole wheat noodles and pasta	White bread
Bulgur		Regular pasta
Popcorn		White rice
Rice cakes		
Brown rice		
Quinoa		

Fresh Vegetables

Vegetables are the richest source of fiber, vitamins, potassium, and magnesium. You can have them whenever and in whatever quantity you want.

What to Eat	What to avoid
All seasonal and fresh vegetables	Regular canned vegetables
Low sodium canned vegetables	

Fruits and Berries

The fruits and berries have the same imperative benefits as vegetables. They are rich in minerals and vitamins. The fruits and berries are low-fat content. They are a good replacement for desserts and snacks. Fruit peels have the highest amount of fiber and nutrients in comparison with fruit flesh.

What to Eat	Eat Occasionally	What to Avoid
All fresh fruits and berries such as apple, pineapple, strawberries, etc	Citrus fruits	Canned fruits Coconut

Dairy

Dairy products are the main source of vitamin D and calcium. The only limit for the dash diet is saturated and high-fat dairy food. You can replace dairy products with nut, almond, cashew, and soy milk.

What to Eat	Eat Occasionally	What to Avoid
Low-fat or fat-free cheese	Low-fat cream	Full-fat cream
Low-fat or fat-free yogurt	Low-fat buttermilk	Full-fat milk
Low-fat or fat-free milk		Full-fat cheese
Low-fat or fat-free skim milk		Full-fat yogurt
Low-fat or fat-free frozen yogurt		

Meat and Poultry

Meat is rich in B vitamins, protein, zinc, and iron. You can have meat in all different styles and varieties. You can broil, grill, bake, or roast it. Make sure not to eat skin and fat from poultry and meat.

What to Eat	Eat Occasionally	What to Avoid
Skinless chicken	Lean cuts of red meat (pork, beef, veal, lamb)	Fat cuts of meat
Chicken fillet	Eggs	Pork belly
		Bacon
		Fat

Fish and Seafood

Fish, which is high in omega-3 fatty acids, is beneficial. All types of seafood and fish are allowed on the dash diet but choose wisely with high omega-3.

What to Eat	What to avoid
Salmon	High sodium canned fish and seafood
Herring	

Nuts, Seeds, and Legumes

Nuts, seeds, and legumes are rich in fiber, phytochemicals, potassium, magnesium, and proteins. They help to fight cancer and cardiovascular disease. They are high in calories and should be eaten in moderation.

What to Eat
All types of seeds
All types of nuts
All types of legumes

Fats and Oils

The main function of dietary fat is to help in absorbing vitamins. High amounts of fat can lead to increased heart disease, obesity, and diabetes.
According to the dash diet, your daily meal plan shouldn't include more than 30 percent of daily calories from fat.

What to Eat	Eat Occasionally	What to Avoid
Margarine	Low-fat	Butter
Vegetable	mayonnaise	Lard
oils	Light salad	Solid
	dressings	shortening

Sweets

You don't have to cut sweets out of your daily diet, but there are some restrictions on the Dash diet.

- Choose sugar-free, low-fat/fat-free sweets
- Replace dessert with fruits and berries

What to Eat	Eat Occasionally	What to Avoid
Fruit/berries	Hard candy	Biscuits
sorbets	Aspartame (NutraSweet,	Crackers
Fruit ice	Equal)	Cookies
Graham crackers	Agave syrup	Soda
Honey	Maple syrup	Unrefined
Sugar-free fruit		sugar
jelly		Table sugar
		Sweet junk
		food

Alcohol and Caffeine

Limit alcohol to two drinks per day for men and one for women. Alcohol and caffeine intake may be restricted by a doctor.

Best Tips for the Dash Diet

- **Physical activity and walking is vital**

  Exercising and walking will enhance the effect of the Dash diet and will help in weight loss too. To stabilize the blood pressure, the perfect combo is a minimum of two hours of walking and 30minutesof exercise per week.

- **Avoid drastic life changes**

  Avoid stressing your body by suddenly changing your eating habits. Go step-by-step until your body adjusts to the new diet.

- **Keep a food journal**

  Keeping a food journal will help you control your food intake and make significant changes in your attitude to food.

- **Make green your compulsory meal partner**

  Make a rule to add green vegetables to every meal. This will provide fiber and potassium.

- **Become a vegetarian**

  Limiting your meat consumption is a very healthy option. Start eating meat no more than once per week. Instead, eat beans, nuts, tofu, and other protein-rich foods.

- **Fresh box in your kitchen**

  Make a fresh box with fruits, vegetables, and rice cakes for snacks. This will help you to resist the temptation of high-sodium junk food.

- **Reading food labels is useful**

  Always read the nutrition labels before buying processed food. Keep in mind that low-sodium canned food must have less than 140mg of sodium per serving.

- **Add spices to life**

  Spices such as rosemary, cayenne pepper, chili pepper, cilantro, dill, cinnamon, etc. can enhance the flavor and appeal of your low-salt meals.

- **Give yourself good snack choices**

  Different types of snacks appeal to different people. It can be a difficult step to switch completely to healthy food. That's why it helps to make a list of your favorite snacks. The food list will change as you get rid of all junk food from your diet.

- **Get a physical examination every two months**

  Some health problems can't be changed by diet alone. Getting a doctor's advice is important. Go in for a physical before starting a diet and then consult a doctor every two months to keep yourself on track and maintain control of your health.

BREAKFAST

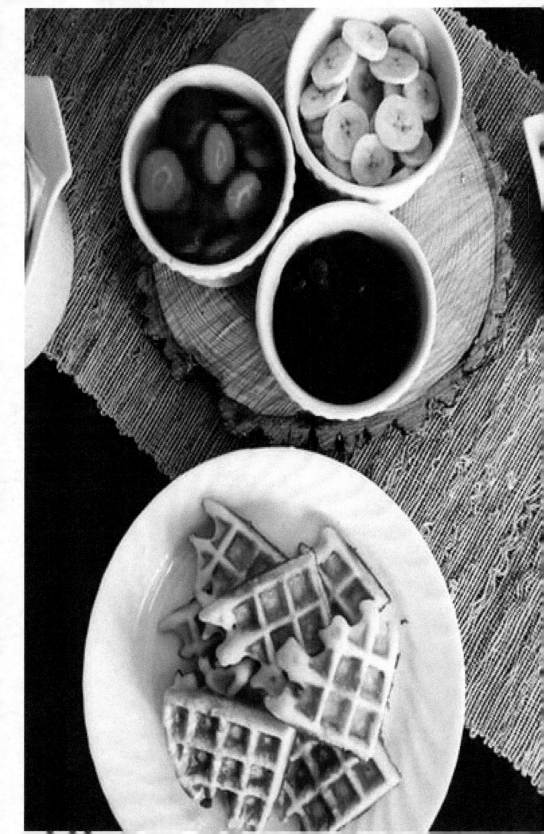

Raspberry Smoothie

2 Servings

Preparation Time: 10 minutes

Ingredients

- 2 cups frozen blueberries
- 2-4 drops liquid stevia
- 1/3 CUPS unsweetened almond milk
- 2 tablespoons unsweetened protein powder.
- Quarter cup fat-free plain Greek yogurt

Directions:

- In a blender, add frozen blueberries and pulse for about 1 minute.
- Add protein powder, stevia almond milk, and yogurt and pulse until desired consistency is achieved.
- Pour the mixture into 2 serving bowls evenly.
- Serve with the topping of your favorite fruit.

Spinach Smoothie Bowl

2 Servings

Preparation Time: 10 minutes

Ingredients

- Half cup avocado, peeled, pitted, and chopped.
- 1 cup fresh baby spinach
- 1 teaspoon fresh lime zest
- Half teaspoons organic vanilla extract
- ¾ cup unsweetened coconut milk
- 2 tablespoons of fresh lime juice.
- 1 teaspoon fresh lime zest
- 4-6 drops liquid stevia

Directions:

- In a blender, add all ingredients and pulse until desired consistency is achieved.
- Pour the mixture into 2 serving bowls evenly.
- Serve with the topping of your favorite fruit.

Yogurt with Granola in a Bowl

4 Servings

Preparation Time: 10 minutes

Ingredients

- 2 cups fat-free plain Greek yogurt
- Half cup oats granola
- 2 tablespoons unsalted walnuts, chopped.
- Half cup fresh blueberries
- 1 large banana peeled and sliced.

Directions:

In a bowl, add yogurt, blueberries, and granola and gently stir to combine.

Divide yogurt mixture into 4 serving bowls.

- Top with banana slices and walnuts and serve.

Apple Oats with Maple syrup

6 Servings

Preparation time: 25 minutes

Ingredients:

- ¼ cup maple syrup
- 2 apples, cored, peeled, and chopped
- ½ teaspoon cinnamon powder
- 1 cup steel-cut oats
- 1 and ½ cups almond milk
- 1 cup non-fat yogurt

Directions:

- In a pot, combine the oats with the milk and the other ingredients except for the yogurt, mix, bring to a simmer and cook over medium-high heat for 15 minutes.
- Divide the yogurt into bowls, divide the apples and oats mix on top and serve for breakfast.

Sweet and Sour Pomegranate Oats

6 Servings

Preparation time: 30 minutes

Ingredients:

- 1 mango, peeled and cubed
- ½ teaspoon vanilla extract
- 3 tablespoons pomegranate seeds
- 3 cups almond milk
- 1 cup steel-cut oats
- 1 tablespoon cinnamon powder

Directions:

- Put the milk in a pot and heat it up over medium heat.
- Add the oats, cinnamon, and the other ingredients, toss, simmer for 20 minutes, divide into bowls and serve for breakfast.

Chia Oats Bowls

6 Servings

Preparation time: 30 minutes

Ingredients:

- ¼ cup pomegranate seeds
- 4 tablespoons chia seeds
- 1 teaspoon vanilla extract
- ½ cup steel cut oats
- 2 cups almond milk

Directions:

- Put the milk in a pot, bring to a simmer over medium heat, add the oats and the other ingredients bring to a simmer, and cook for 20 minutes.
- Divide the mix into bowls and serve for breakfast.

Red Carrots Hash

6 Servings

Preparation time: 30 minutes

Ingredients:

- 1 cup low-fat cheddar cheese, shredded
- 8 eggs, whisked
- 1 cup coconut milk
- A pinch of salt and black pepper
- 2 carrots, peeled and cubed
- 1 tablespoon olive oil
- 1 yellow onion, chopped

Directions:

- Heat up a pan with the oil over medium heat, add the onion and the carrots, toss, and brown for 5 minutes.
- Add the eggs and the other ingredients, toss, cook for 15 minutes, often stirring, divide between plates and serve.

Spring Omelet with red pepper

6 Servings

Preparation time: 25 minutes

Ingredients:

- 1 tablespoon olive oil
- 1 cup red bell peppers, chopped
- 4 spring onions, chopped
- ¾ cup low-fat cheese, shredded
- 4 eggs, whisked
- A pinch of black pepper
- ¼ cup low-sodium bacon, chopped

Directions:

- Heat up a pan with the oil over medium heat, add the spring onions and the bell peppers, mix and cook for 5 minutes.
- Add the eggs and the other ingredients, toss, spread into the pan, cook for 5 minutes, flip, cook for another 5 minutes, divide between plates and serve.

Low-Fat Cheese Frittata

6 Servings

Preparation time: 30 minutes

Ingredients:

- 1 tablespoon low-fat cheese, shredded
- 1 red onion, chopped
- 1 tablespoon olive oil
- A pinch of black pepper
- 4 eggs, whisked
- 2 tablespoons parsley, chopped

Directions:

- Heat up a pan with the oil over medium heat, add the onion and the black pepper, stir and sauté for 5 minutes.
- Add the eggs mixed with the other ingredients, spread into the pan, introduce in the oven, and cook at 360 degrees F for 15 minutes.
- Divide the frittata between plates and serve.

Baked Black Beans

10 Servings

Preparation time: 40 minutes

Ingredients:

- 4 ounces canned black beans, no-salt-added, drained and rinsed
- ½ cup green onions, chopped
- 1 cup low-fat mozzarella cheese, shredded
- Cooking spray
- 8 eggs, whisked
- 2 red onions, chopped
- 1 red bell pepper, chopped

Directions:

- Grease a baking pan with the cooking spray and spread the black beans, onions, green onions, and bell pepper into the pan.

- Add the eggs mixed with the cheese, introduce in the oven and bake at 380 degrees F for 30 minutes.
- Divide the mix between plates and serve for breakfast.

LUNCH

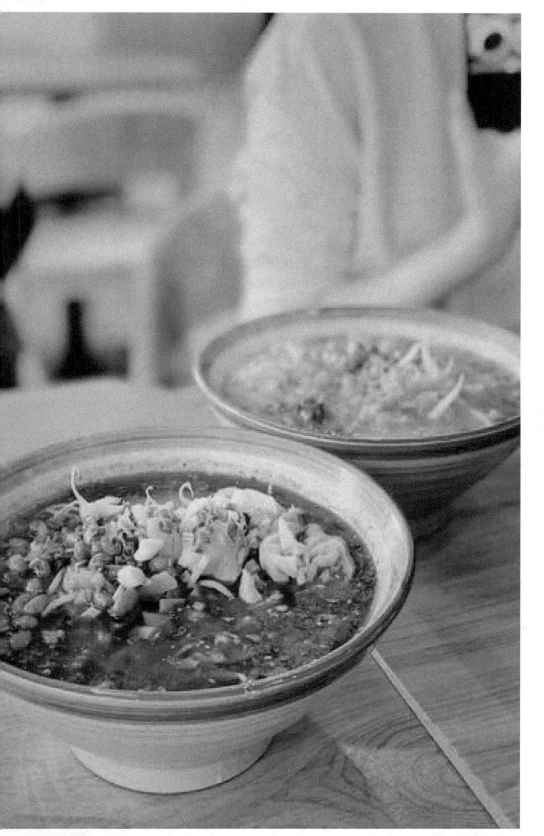

Beef Tenderloin with Rosemary

10Servings

Preparation Time: 60 minutes

Ingredients

- 1 (3-lb.) center-cut beef tenderloin roast, trimmed.
- 1 tablespoon of fresh rosemary minced and divided.
- Freshly ground black pepper, to taste
- 4 garlic cloves, minced.
- Pinch of salt
- 2 tablespoons olive oil

Directions:

- Preheat the oven to 425 °F.
- Grease a large shallow roasting pan.
- Place beef into the prepared roasting pan.
- Rub the beef with garlic, rosemary, salt, and black pepper and drizzle with oil.
- Roast the beef for about 45-50 minutes.

- Remove from the oven and place the roast onto a cutting board for about 10 minutes.
- With a sharp knife, cut beef tenderloin into desired-sized slices and serve.

Lemony Steak

4 Servings

Preparation Time: 22 minutes

Ingredients

- 2 teaspoons fresh lemon juice
- Pinch of salt
- 1 lb. flank steak, trimmed.
- 2halftablespoons extra-virgin olive oil, divided.
- Freshly ground black pepper, to taste

Directions:

- In a large bowl, mix the lemon juice, 1halfteaspoons of extra-virgin olive oil, salt, and black pepper.
- Add steak and coat with mixture generously.
- In a non-stick skillet, heat the remaining oil over medium-high heat and cook the steak for 5-6 minutes per side.
- Pour the steak onto a cutting board for about 10 minutes before slicing.

- With a sharp knife, cut the beef steak into desired-sized slices diagonally across the grain and serve.

Fresh Green Peas and Cauliflower Curry

3 Servings

Preparation Time: 30 minutes

Ingredients

- 2 medium tomatoes, chopped.
- 2 tablespoons olive oil
- Half tablespoons fresh ginger, minced.
- 1 teaspoon ground coriander
- Quarter teaspoons ground turmeric
- 1 CUPS fresh green peas, shelled.
- Freshly ground black pepper, to taste
- Quarter cup water
- 3 garlic cloves, minced.
- 1 teaspoon ground cumin
- 1 teaspoon cayenne pepper
- 2 CUPS cauliflower, chopped.
- Pinch of salt
- Half cup warm water

Directions:

- In a blender, add tomato and quarter cup of water and pulse until a smooth puree forms.
- Set aside.
- In a large skillet, heat the oil over medium heat and sauté the garlic, ginger, green chilies, and spices for about 1 minute.
- Add the cauliflower, peas, and tomato puree and cook, stirring for about 3-4 minutes.
- Add the warm water and bring to a boil.
- Reduce the heat to medium-low and cook, covered for about 8-10 minutes or until vegetables are done completely. Serve hot.

Nutty and Crunchy Veggie Loaf

6 Servings

Preparation Time: 1 hour and 45 minutes

Ingredients

- Half tablespoons olive oil

- 1 teaspoon dried rosemary, crushed.

- ¾ cup pecans, chopped.

- 3 cups whole-wheat breadcrumbs

- Pinch of salt

- Half cup celery stalk, chopped.

- 1 teaspoon dried basil, crushed.

- ¾ cup unsalted walnuts, chopped.

- 2 ½ unsweetened soy milk

- Freshly ground black pepper, to taste

Directions:

- Preheat the oven to 350 degrees F.

- Lightly, grease a loaf pan.

- In a large bowl, add all the ingredients and mix until well combined.

- Pour the mixture into the prepared loaf pan.

- Bake for about 60-90 minutes or until the top becomes golden brown.

- Remove from the oven and place the loaf pan onto a wire rack for about 10 minutes.

- Carefully, invert the loaf onto a platter. Cut into desired-sized slices and serve.

Spinach with chickpeas Stew

4 Servings

Preparation Time: 45 minutes

Ingredients

- 1 tablespoon olive oil

- 2 cups carrots peeled and chopped.

- 1 teaspoon red pepper flake

- 2 cups low-sodium vegetable broth

- 2 cups fresh spinach, chopped.

- 1 medium onion, chopped.

- 2 garlic cloves, minced.

- 2 large tomatoes, chopped. finely

- 2 cups cooked chickpeas

- 1 tablespoon fresh lemon juice

Directions:

- In a large pan, heat oil over medium heat and sauté the onion and carrot for about 6 minutes.

- Stir in the garlic and red pepper flakes and sauté for about 1 minute.

- Add the tomatoes and cook for about 2-3 minutes.
- Add the broth and bring to a boil.
- Reduce the heat to low and simmer for about 10 minutes.
- Stir in the chickpeas and simmer for about 5 minutes.
- Stir in the spinach and simmer for 3-4 minutes more.
- Stir in the lemon juice and remove from the heat. Serve hot.

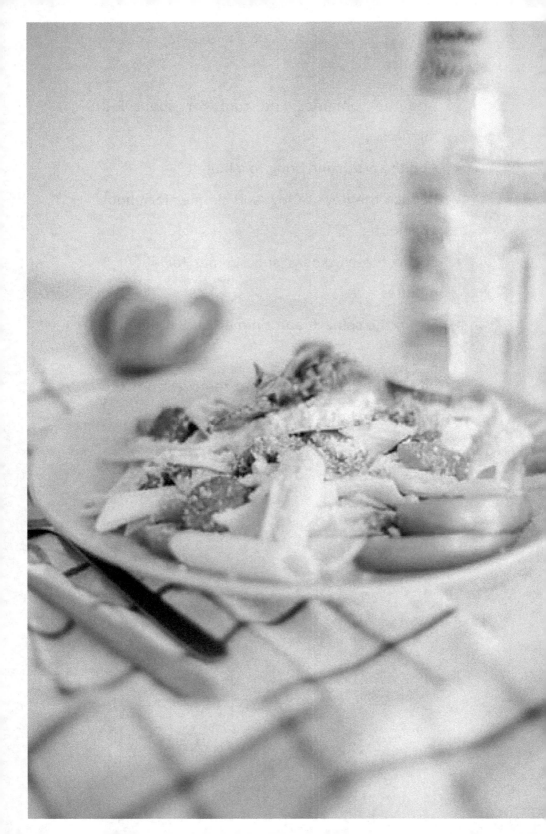

Lentils and Quinoa Stew

6 Servings

Preparation Time: 45 minutes

Ingredients

- 1 tablespoon olive oil
- 3 celery stalks, chopped.
- 4 garlic cloves, minced.
- Half cup dried quinoa rinsed.
- 1 teaspoon red chili powder
- 2 cups fresh spinach, chopped.
- 3 carrots peeled and chopped.
- 1 yellow onion, chopped.
- 4 cups tomatoes, chopped.
- 1 cup red lentils, rinsed.
- 5 cups low-sodium vegetable broth

Directions:

- In a large pan, heat the oil over medium heat and sauté the celery, onion, and carrot for about 4-5 minutes.
- Add the garlic and sauté for about 1 minute.

- Add the remaining ingredients except for the spinach and bring to a boil.

- Reduce the heat to low and simmer covered for about 20 minutes.

- Stir in spinach and simmer for about 3-4 minutes. Serve hot.

Gingery Turkey Mix

6 Servings

Preparation time: 30 minutes

Ingredients:

- 2 tablespoons olive oil
- 1 teaspoon ginger, grated
- A pinch of black pepper
- 1 cup low-sodium vegetable stock
- 1 turkey breast, boneless, skinless, and roughly cubed
- 2 scallions, chopped
- 1 pound bok choy, torn

Directions:

- Heat up a pot with the oil over medium-high heat; add the scallions and the ginger and sauté for 2 minutes.
- Add the meat and brown for 5 minutes more.

- Add the rest of the ingredients, toss, simmer for 13 minutes more, divide between plates and serve.

Chicken Chives

6 Servings

Preparation time: 35 minutes

Ingredients:

- 1½ cup low-sodium vegetable stock
- A pinch of black pepper
- 1 ½tablespoon cilantro, chopped
- 1½ tablespoon chives, chopped
- 3 chicken breasts, skinless, boneless, and roughly cubed
- 3 red onions, sliced
- 2 tablespoons olive oil

Directions:

- Heat up a pan with the oil over medium heat, add the onions and a pinch of black pepper, and sauté for 10 minutes, stirring often.
- Add the chicken and cook for 3 minutes more.
- Add the rest of the ingredients, bring to a simmer and cook over medium heat for 12 minutes more.
- Divide the chicken and onions, mix between plates and serve.

Peppery Turkey and Rice

6 Servings

Preparation time: 52 minutes

Ingredients:

- 2 small Serrano peppers, chopped
- 2 garlic cloves, minced
- 3 tablespoons olive oil
- ½ red bell pepper chopped
- A pinch of black pepper
- ½ turkey breast, skinless, boneless, and cubed
- 1½ cup brown rice
- 2 cups low-sodium vegetable stock
- 1½ teaspoon hot paprika

Directions:

- Heat up a pan with the oil over medium heat, add the Serrano peppers and garlic and sauté for 2 minutes.
- Add the meat and brown it for 5 minutes.
- Add the rice and the other ingredients, bring to a simmer, and cook over medium heat for 35 minutes.
- Stir, divide between plates, and serve.

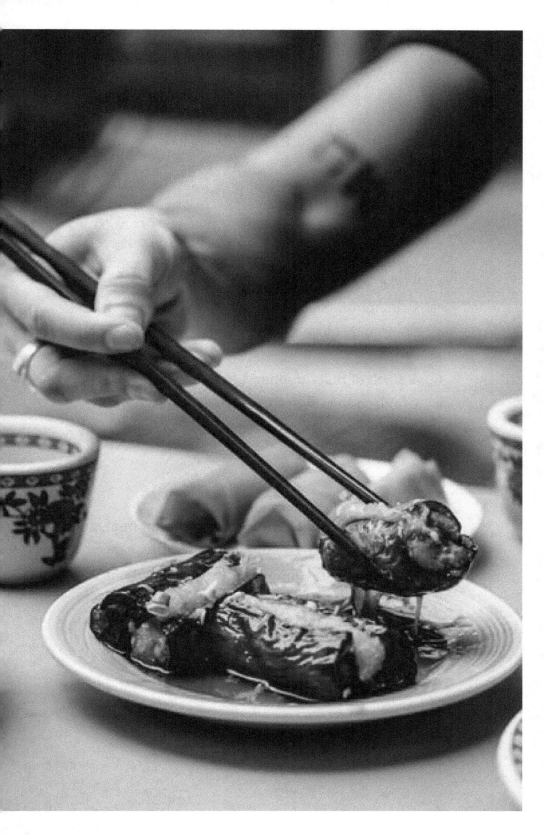

Leeks with Chicken

6 Servings

Preparation time: 50 minutes

Ingredients:

- 1 cup low-sodium vegetable stock
- 5 leek, roughly chopped
- 1 cup lemon juice
- 1½ pound chicken breast, skinless, boneless, and cubed
- A pinch of black pepper
- 2 tablespoons avocado oil
- 1 tablespoon tomato sauce, no-salt-added

Directions:

- Heat up a pan with the oil over medium heat, add the leeks, toss and sauté for 10 minutes.
- Add the chicken and the other ingredients, toss, cook over medium heat for 20 minutes more, divide between plates and serve.

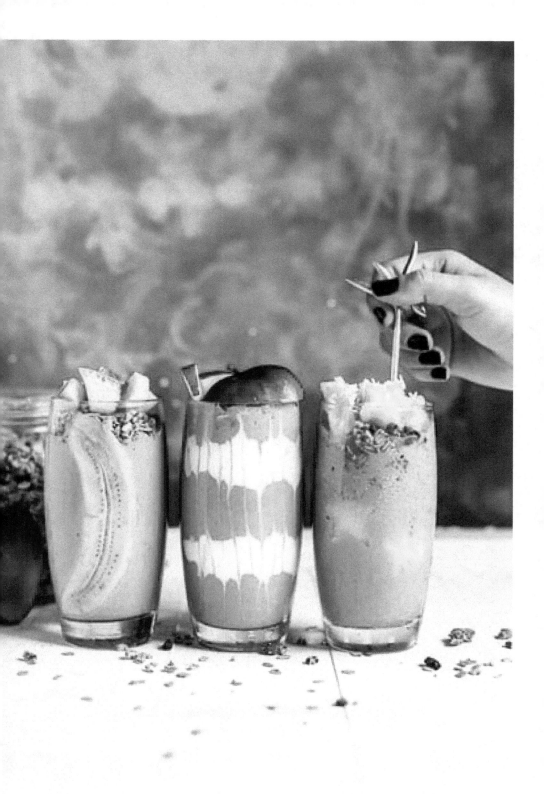

JUICE AND SMOOTHIES

Spiced Pumpkin Smoothie

2 Servings

Preparation Time: 10 minutes

Ingredients

- 1 cup homemade pumpkin puree
- 1 teaspoon ground flaxseed
- 1half cup unsweetened almond milk
- 1 medium banana peeled and sliced.
- Quarter teaspoons ground cinnamon
- Quarter cup ice cubes

Directions:

- In a high-speed blender, add all ingredients and pulse until smooth.
- Pour into 2 serving glasses and serve immediately.

Green Smoothie with Cucumber

2 Servings

Preparation Time: 10 minutes

Ingredients

- 1 small cucumber peeled and chopped.
- Half cup lettuce, torn.
- Quarter cup fresh mint leaves
- 1 teaspoon fresh lemon juice
- Quarter cup ice cubes
- 2 cups mixed fresh greens.
- Quarter cup fresh parsley leaves
- 2-3 drops liquid stevia
- 1 ½ cups filtered water

Directions:

- In a high-speed blender, add all ingredients and pulse until smooth.
- Pour into 2 serving glasses and serve immediately.

Avocado Smoothie with Chocolate

2 Servings

Preparation Time: 18 minutes

Ingredients

- 1 medium avocado, peeled, pitted, and chopped.
- Half teaspoons organic vanilla extract
- Quarter cup ice cubes
- 1 small banana peeled and sliced.
- 3 tablespoons cacao powder
- 1¾ cups chilled fat-free milk

Directions:

- In a high-speed blender, add all ingredients and pulse until smooth.
- Pour into 2 serving glasses and serve immediately.

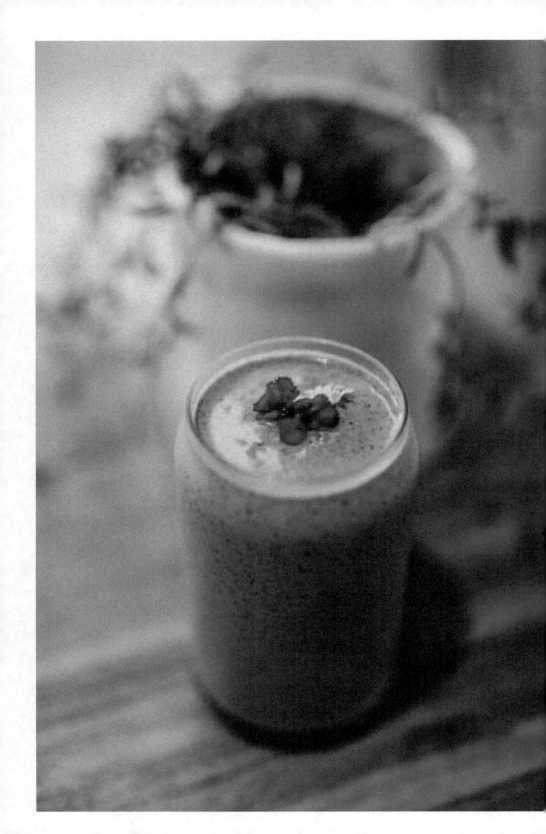

Silky Avocado & Spinach Smoothie

2 Servings

Preparation Time: 10 minutes

Ingredients

- 2 cups fresh baby spinach
- 1 tablespoon hemp seed
- 3-4 drops liquid stevia
- Half of the avocado, peeled, pitted, and chopped.
- half teaspoon ground cinnamon
- 2 cups chilled filtered water

Directions:

- In a high-speed blender, add all ingredients and pulse until smooth.
- Pour into 2 serving glasses and serve immediately.

Yummy Strawberry Juice

4 serving

Preparation time: 10 minutes

Ingredients

- 4 tsp. fresh lime juice
- 8CUP chilled filtered water
- 8CUP fresh strawberries, hulled

Directions

- Take a blender and add all ingredients, and pulse well. Through a strainer, strain the juice and transfer it into two glasses. Serve and enjoy

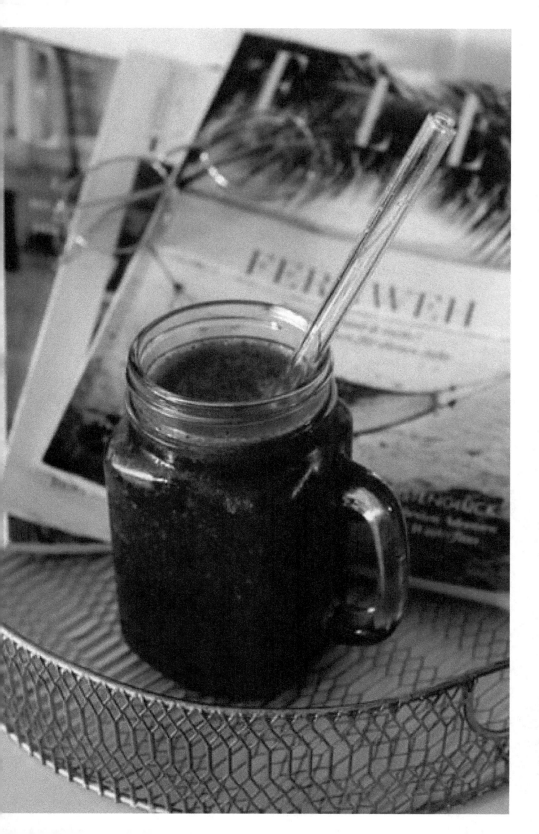

Tangy Kiwi Juice

4 Serves

Preparation time: 10 minutes

Ingredients

- 8CUP chilled filtered water
- 8 medium kiwis, peeled and chopped

Directions

- In a blender, place kiwi and water and pulse well. Through a strainer, strain the juice and transfer it into 2 glasses, and serve immediately.

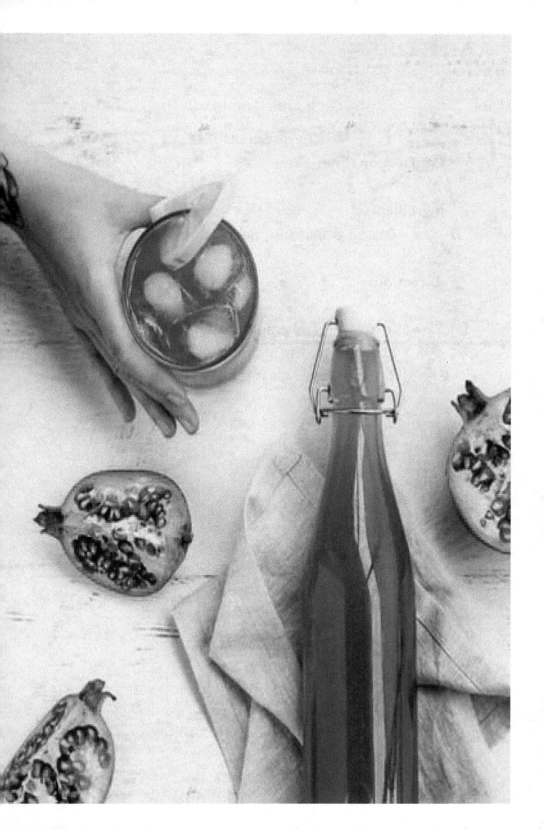

Delicious Grapefruit Juice

4 Serves

Preparation time: 10 minutes

Ingredients

- 8 large grapefruits, peeled and sectioned

Directions

- In a juicer, add grapefruit and extract the juice according to the manufacturer's directions. Transfer into 2 glasses and serve immediately.

Refreshing Orange Juice

4 Serving

Preparation time: 10 minutes

Ingredients
- Pinch of ground black pepper
- 12 medium oranges, peeled and sectioned

Directions

- In a juicer, add orange pieces and extract the juice according to the manufacturer's directions. Transfer into 2 glasses and stir in black pepper. Serve immediately.

Apple & Pomegranate Juice

4 Serving

Preparation time: 10 minutes

Ingredients

- 4 tsp. fresh lemon juice
- 4 large apples, cored and sliced
- Pinch of ground black pepper
- 6 cups fresh pomegranate seeds

Directions

- In a juicer, add all ingredients and extract the juice according to the manufacturer's directions. Transfer into 2 glasses and serve immediately.

DINNER

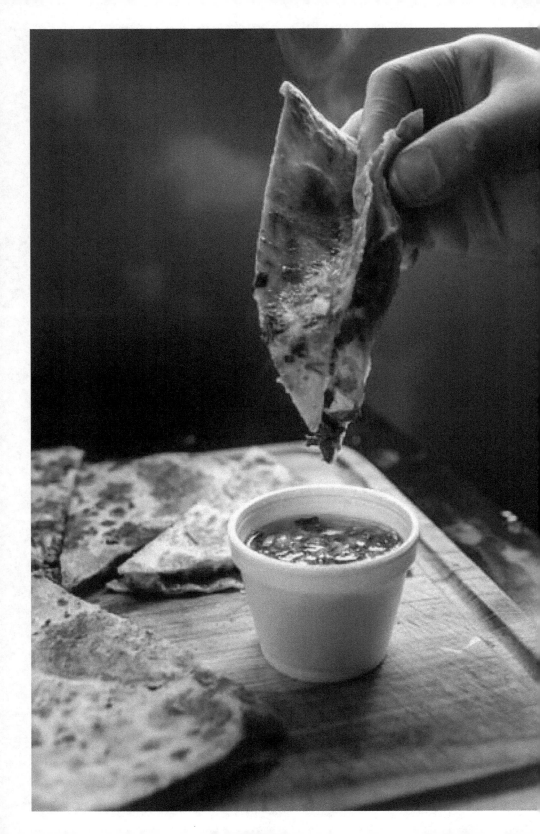

Veggies Stuffed Steak

6 Servings

Preparation Time: 55 minutes

Ingredients

- 1.5-lb. flank steak
- Freshly ground black pepper, to taste
- 2 small garlic cloves, minced.
- 1 medium green bell pepper seeded and chopped.
- Pinch of salt
- 1 tablespoon olive oil
- 6 oz. fresh spinach, chopped. finely
- 1 medium tomato, chopped. finely

Directions:

- Preheat the oven to 425 °F. Grease a large baking dish.
- Place flank steak onto a smooth surface.
- Hold a sharp knife parallel to the work surface, slice the steak horizontally, without cutting all

the way through, that you can open like a book.

- With a meat mallet, flatten the steak into an even thickness.
- Sprinkle the steak with salt and black pepper evenly.
- In a skillet, heat the oil over medium heat and sauté the garlic for about 1 minute.
- Add the spinach and black pepper and cook for about 2 minutes.
- Stir in bell pepper and tomato and immediately remove from the heat.
- Pour the spinach mixture into a bowl and set aside to cool slightly.
- Place the filling on the top of the steak evenly.
- Roll up the steak to seal the filling.
- With cotton twine, tie the steak.
- Place the steak roll into the prepared baking dish.
- Bake for about 30-35 minutes.

- Remove from oven and set aside to cool slightly. With a sharp knife, cut the roll in desired-sized slices and serve.

Green Onions Cod Mix

6 Servings

Preparation time: 30 minutes

Ingredients:

- 1½ tablespoon olive oil
- 1 tablespoon lemon juice
- 1 cup green onion, chopped
- 4 cod fillets, boneless
- 1 cup low-fat parmesan cheese, shredded
- 3 garlic cloves, minced

Directions:

- Heat a pan with the oil over medium heat, add the garlic and the green onions, toss and sauté for 5 minutes.
- Add the fish and cook it for 4 minutes on each side.
- Add the lemon juice, sprinkle the parmesan on top, cook everything for 2 minutes more, divide between plates and serve.

Lemony Chives Tilapia

6 Servings

Preparation time: 25 minutes

Ingredients:

- 3 teaspoons lemon zest, grated
- 2 red onions, roughly chopped
- 3 tablespoons chives, chopped
- 4 tilapia fillets, boneless
- 3 tablespoons olive oil
- 1 ½ tablespoon lemon juice

Directions:

- Heat a pan with the oil over medium heat, add the onions, lemon zest, and lemon juice, toss and sauté for 5 minutes.
- Add the fish and the chives, cook for 5 minutes on each side, divide between plates and serve.

Tarragon Roast

6 Servings

Preparation time: 8 hours 10 minutes

Ingredients:

- 2 shallots, chopped
- 1½ cup low-sodium vegetable stock
- 1½ tablespoon thyme, chopped
- 1½ tablespoon mustard
- 2 pounds pork roast, sliced
- 3 tablespoons olive oil
- Black pepper to the taste
- 1½ tablespoon tarragon, chopped

Directions:

- In a slow cooker, combine the roast with the black pepper and the other ingredients, put the lid on, and cook on Low for 8 hours.
- Divide the pork roast between plates, drizzle the mustard sauce all over and serve.

Pork with nutty Capers

6 Servings

Preparation time: 45 minutes

Ingredients:

- 1½ cup bean sprouts
- 1 yellow onion, cut into wedges
- Black pepper to the taste
- 3 tablespoons olive oil
- 1½ cup low-sodium vegetable stock
- 3 tablespoons capers, drained
- 1 pound pork chops

Directions:

- Heat a pan with the oil over medium-high heat, add the onion and the meat, and brown for 5 minutes.

- Add the rest of the ingredients, introduce the pan in the oven, and bake at 390 degrees F for 30 minutes.
- Divide everything between plates and serve

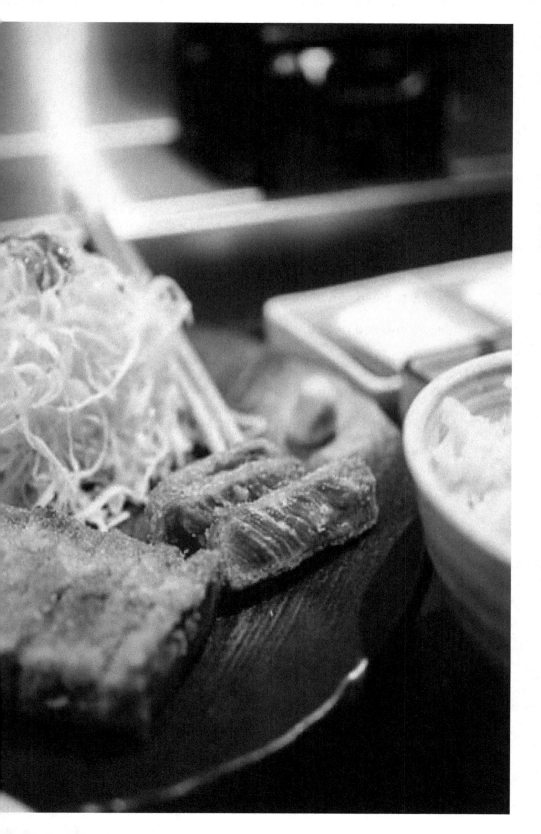

Green Beans with Pork

6 Servings

Preparation time: 30 minutes

Ingredients:

- Black pepper to the taste
- 1 tablespoon olive oil
- 1 cup red hot chili pepper, chopped
- 1 cup low-sodium vegetable stock
- 1 yellow onion, chopped
- 2 pounds pork meat, cut into strips
- 1½ pound green beans, trimmed and halved
- 1 red bell pepper, chopped

Directions:

- Heat a pan with the oil over medium-high heat, add the onion and sauté for 5 minutes.
- Add the meat and brown for 5 minutes more.

- Add the rest of the ingredients, toss, cook for 10 minutes over medium heat, divide between plates and serve.

Classical Mushroom Stew

4 Servings

Preparation Time: 30 minutes

Ingredients

- 2 tablespoons olive oil
- 3 garlic cloves, minced.
- Quarter lb. fresh shiitake mushrooms, chopped.
- Freshly ground black pepper, to taste
- Half cup unsweetened coconut milk
- 2 onions, chopped.
- Half lb. fresh button mushrooms, chopped.
- Quarter lb. fresh Portobello mushrooms, chopped.
- quarter cup low-sodium vegetable broth
- 2 tablespoons fresh parsley, chopped.

Directions:

- In a large skillet, heat oil over medium heat and sauté the onion and garlic for 4-5 minutes.

- Add the mushrooms, salt, and black pepper and cook for 4-5 minutes.
- Add the broth and coconut milk and bring to a gentle boil.
- Simmer for 4-5 minutes or until desired doneness.
- Stir in the cilantro and remove from heat. Serve hot.

Bell Pepper and Tofu Stew

6 Servings

Preparation Time: 30 minutes

Ingredients

- 2 tablespoons chile-garlic sauce
- 1 (16-oz.) jar roasted red peppers, rinsed and rinsed.
- 16 oz. extra-firm tofu, drained, pressed, and cubed
- 1 jalapeño pepper seeded and chopped.
- 4 CUPS water
- 2 medium bell peppers seeded and sliced.
- 1 (10-oz.) package frozen baby spinach, thawed.

Directions:

- In a food processor, add chile-garlic sauce, jalapeño pepper, and roasted red peppers and pulse until a smooth puree form.

- In a large pan, mix puree and water over medium-high heat and ring to a boil.

- Add bell peppers and tofu and stir to combine.

- Reduce the heat to medium and cook for about 5 minutes.

- Stir in spinach and cook for about 5 minutes. Serve hot.

DESSERT

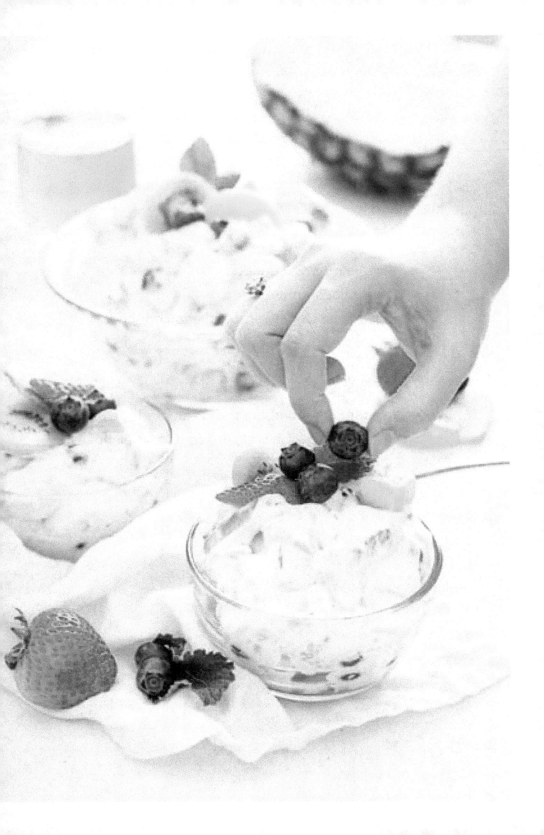

Nutty Almond Cream

6 Servings

Preparation time: 10 minutes

Ingredients:

- 1 teaspoon vanilla extract
- 1 cup almonds, chopped
- 3 cups coconut cream
- 3 peaches, stones removed and chopped

Directions:

- In a blender, combine the cream and the other ingredients, pulse well, divide into small bowls and serve cold.

Sweet Plums

6 Servings

Preparation time: 25 minutes

Ingredients:

- 2 tablespoons coconut sugar
- 1 teaspoon cinnamon powder
- 1 cup of water
- 1½ pound plums, stones removed and halved

Directions:

- In a pan, combine the plums with the sugar and the other ingredients, bring to a simmer and cook over medium heat for 15 minutes.
- Divide into bowls and serve cold.

Chia Apples wedges

6 Servings

Preparation time: 20 minutes

Ingredients:

- 1½ teaspoon vanilla extract
- 3 cups naturally unsweetened apple juice
- 3 cups apples, cored and cut into wedges
- 3 tablespoons chia seeds

Directions:

- In a small pot, combine the apples with the chia seeds and the other ingredients, toss, cook over medium heat for 10 minutes, divide into bowls and serve cold.

SOUPS AND SALADS

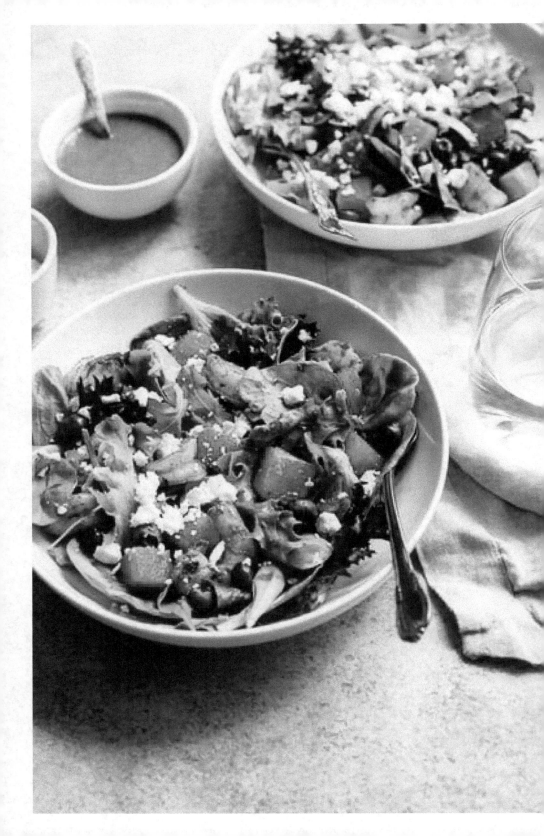

Mixed Veggie Salad

6 Servings

Preparation Time: 20 minutes

Ingredients

- **For Dressing**
    - 1 small avocado, peeled, pitted, and chopped.
    - Quarter cup fat-free plain Greek yogurt
    - 1 garlic clove, chopped.
    - 2 tablespoons fresh parsley.
    - 2 tablespoons of fresh lemon juice.
    - Pinch of salt
- **For Salad**
    - 6 cups fresh spinach, shredded.
    - 2 medium zucchinis cut into thin slices.
    - 1 cup bell pepper seeded and sliced thinly.
    - 1 cup cucumber sliced thinly.
    - ½ cup cherry tomatoes halved.
    - Quarter cup Kalamata olives pitted.

Directions:

- For the dressing: in a food processor, add all the ingredients and pulse until smooth.
- For the salad: in a salad bowl, add all the ingredients and mix well.
- Pour the dressing over salad and gently toss to coat well. Serve immediately.

Moroccan Chickpeas Salad

4 Servings

Preparation Time: 15 minutes

Ingredients

- **For Salad**
    - 2 cups cooked chickpeas
    - 1 head butter lettuce, torn.
    - 1 bell pepper seeded and chopped.
    - 2 cups cherry tomatoes, halved.
    - 1 red onion, chopped.
    - 4 tablespoons fresh cilantro, chopped.
- **For Dressing**
    - 1 Serrano pepper seeded and minced.
    - 1 garlic clove, minced.
    - Quarter cup olive oil
    - 2 tablespoons of fresh lemon juice.
    - Quarter teaspoons red pepper flakes, crushed.
    - Pinch of salt

Directions:

- **For the salad:** in a large bowl, add all ingredients and mix.
- **For the dressing:** in a small bowl, add all ingredients and beat until well combined.
- Add dressing in the bowl of salad and gently toss to coat well. Serve immediately.

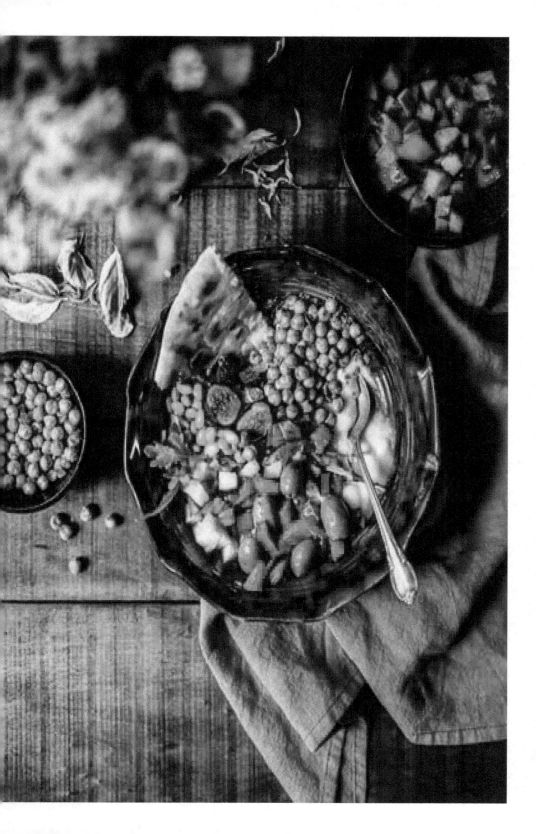

Pomegranate Salad with Kidney Beans

4 Servings

Preparation Time: 10 minutes

Ingredients

- 2 cups cooked white kidney beans.
- Quarter cup scallion greens, chopped. finely
- 1 tablespoon fresh lime juice.
- 1 cup fresh pomegranate seeds
- 2 tablespoons fresh parsley leaves, chopped.
- Pinch of salt

Directions:

- In a large bowl, add all ingredients and toss to coat well.
- Serve immediately.

Cold Zucchini Soup

5 Servings

Preparation Time: 30 minutes

Ingredients

- 2 teaspoons olive oil
- 2 garlic cloves, minced.
- 1 lb. zucchini, sliced.
- 2 tablespoons fresh cilantro, chopped.
- Half cup onion, chopped.
- 1 tablespoon curry powder
- 4 CUPS fat-free milk

Directions:

- In a large pan, heat oil over medium-high heat and sauté onion for about 4-6 minutes.
- Add garlic and curry powder and sauté for about 1 minute.
- Add zucchini and cook for about 2-3 minutes.
- Reduce the heat to medium and cook for about 4-5 minutes.
- Remove from heat and let it cool slightly.

- In a blender, add zucchini mixture and milk in batches and pulse until a chunky mixture forms.
- Pour the mixture into a bowl and refrigerate to chill completely.
- Serve with the garnishing of cilantro.

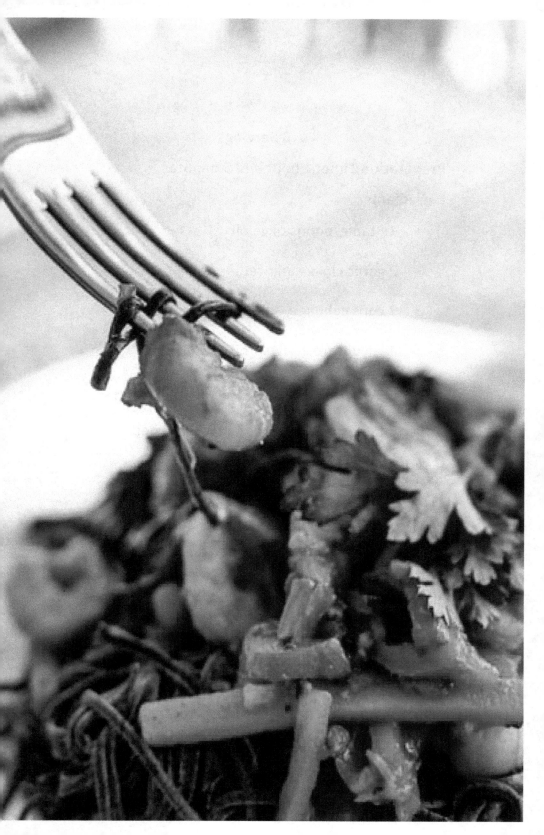

Chickpeas with Beef Soup

6 Servings

Preparation Time: 1 hour and 5 minutes

Ingredients

- 1.5 tablespoons olive oil

- 2 garlic cloves, minced.

- 3 cups cabbage, shredded.

- 1 ½ cups fresh mushrooms, sliced.

- 6 cups low-sodium chicken broth

- 2 tablespoons fresh cilantro, chopped.

- ¾ cup onion, chopped.

- 1 lb. lean ground beef

- ½ cup bell peppers seeded and chopped.

- Quarter cup tomatoes, chopped.

- 2 tablespoons fresh lemon juice

- Freshly ground black pepper, to taste

Directions:

- In a large soup pan, heat oil over medium heat and sauté onion for about 3-4 minutes.

- Add garlic and sauté for about 1 minute.

- Add beef and cook for about 4-5 minutes.

- Add vegetables and cook for abbot 4-5 minutes.

- Add chickpeas and broth and bring to a boil.

- Reduce the heat to low and simmer, covered for about 25-30 minutes.

- Stir in lemon juice, cilantro and black pepper and remove from the heat. Serve hot.

Ground Beef with mushroom Soup

6 Servings

Preparation Time: 45 minutes

Ingredients

- 1 tablespoon olive oil
- Half lb. fresh mushrooms, sliced.
- 1 garlic clove, minced.
- 6 cups low-sodium chicken broth
- Freshly ground black pepper, to taste
- 1 lb. lean ground beef
- 1 small yellow onion, chopped.
- 1 lb. head bok choy, stalks, and leaves separated and chopped.

Directions:

- In a large pan, heat oil over medium-high heat and cook the beef for about 5 minutes.
- Add the onion, mushrooms and garlic and cook for about 5 minutes.
- Add the bok choy stalks and cook for about 4-5 minutes.

- Add broth and bring to a boil. Reduce the heat to low and simmer, covered for about 10 minutes.
- Stir in the bok choy leaves and cook for about 5 minutes.
- Stir in black pepper and serve hot.

Veggie and Salmon Soup

4 Servings

Preparation Time: 45 minutes

Ingredients

- 2 tablespoons olive oil

- 2 garlic cloves, minced.

- 1 Chinese head cabbage, chopped.

- 5 cups low-sodium vegetable broth

- Quarter cup fresh cilantro, minced.

- Freshly ground black pepper, to taste

- 1 shallot, chopped.

- 1 jalapeño pepper, chopped.

- 2 small bell peppers seeded and chopped.

- 2 (4-oz.) boneless salmon fillets, cubed.

- 2 tablespoons fresh lemon juice

Directions:

- In a large soup pan, heat oil over medium heat and sauté shallot and garlic for about 2-3 minutes.

- Add cabbage and bell peppers and sauté for about 3-4 minutes.
- Add broth and bring to a boil over high heat.
- Reduce the heat to medium-low and simmer for about 10 minutes.
- Add salmon and cook for about 5-6 minutes.
- Stir in the cilantro, lemon juice, and black pepper and cook for about 1-2 minutes. Serve hot.

Fresh Apple Salad

4 Servings

Preparation Time: 10 minutes

Ingredients

- 4 large apples cored and sliced.
- 3 tablespoons extra-virgin olive oil.
- 6 cups fresh baby spinach
- 2 tablespoons of organic apple cider vinegar.

Directions:

- In a large bowl, add all the ingredients and toss to coat well.
- Serve immediately.

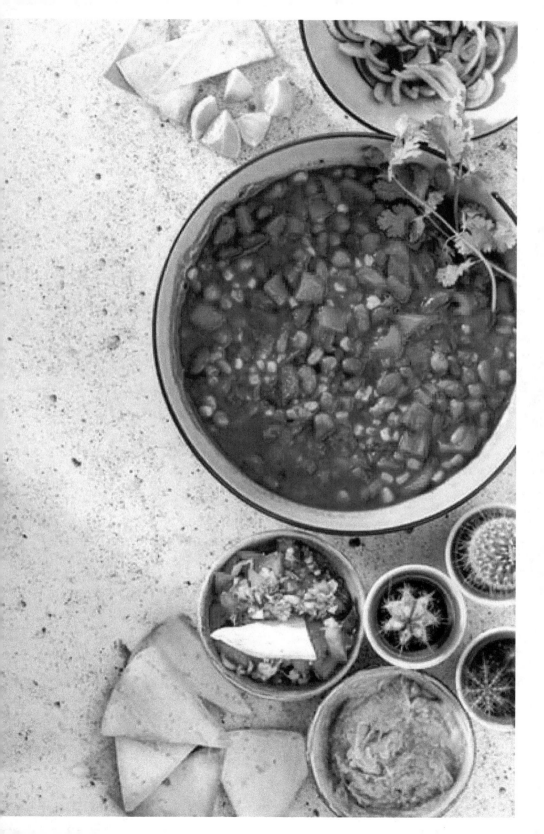

Green Apple & Blueberry Salad

4 Servings

Preparation Time: 15 minutes

Ingredients

- 4 tablespoons fat-free yogurt

- 2 small apples were cored and chopped.

- 1 avocado, peeled, pitted, and chopped.

- Half cup unsalted almonds, slivered.

- 1 tablespoon unsweetened applesauce.

- 1 cup fresh blueberries

- 1 cup unsweetened coconut flakes

Directions:

- **In** a large bowl, add yogurt and applesauce and stir to combine.

- Add remaining ingredients and gently stir to combine.

- Serve immediately.

Tropical bright Fruit Salad

6 Servings

Preparation Time: 15 minutes

Ingredients

- 1 cup fresh pineapple peeled and chopped.
- 1 cup mango, peeled, pitted, and cubed.
- quarter cup dried cranberries
- 2 tablespoons of fresh orange juice.
- Freshly ground black pepper, to taste
- 1 cup papaya peeled and cubed.
- 8 cup fresh baby spinach
- Quarter cup fresh mint leaves, chopped.
- Pinch of salt
- Half cup unsalted almonds, chopped.

Directions:

- In a large salad bowl, add all ingredients except for almonds and toss to coat well.
- Cover and refrigerate to chill before serving.
- Serve with the topping of almonds.

Tangy Orange & Beet Salad

4 Servings

Preparation Time: 10 minutes

Ingredients

- 3 large oranges, peeled, seeded, and sectioned.
- 6 cup fresh rocket
- 3 tablespoons olive oil
- 2 beets, trimmed, peeled, and sliced.
- Quarter cup unsalted walnuts, chopped.
- Pinch of salt

Directions:

- In a salad bowl, place all ingredients and gently toss to coat.
- Serve immediately.